# FROM FAT - FIT
### (Essential and innovative weight-loss advice)

## OSAGIE JERRY E. XAVIER

# DEDICATION

This book is dedicated to my wife (Adesola), family and friends, to whom this book will not be written and to all who want to live a healthy life.

# CONTENTS

# INTRODUCTION

Before the idea of losing weight even entered our society, individuals simply ate whatever their mothers made for supper and went to work. The labor was done on one's feet in the fields or on a warehouse floor, not in front of a computer screen as it is in today's culture. The only way to work, and the reason it was called work, was physically, thus people worked physically. Because they were burning off a lot more calories than they were taking in, folks could frequently eat whatever they wanted at this time.

However, like with all good things, it too has come and gone, and the technology of our modern world has left us in one state—an overweight one. Our comfort levels have multiplied tenfold while our lifestyles have undergone such radical transformation. Every rose has its thorn, as the saying goes, and in our society, our desire for pleasant lifestyles and reduced work hours has started to manifest itself in our expanding waistlines.

The unfortunate aspect of it all is that it gets riskier the more weight you gain. If you don't do anything about your excess weight, it will eventually manifest as illness, whether it be diabetes or a heart condition. Prior to reaching the point when you can no longer control your weight, you must actively prevent weight gain and try to lose it. Being at a healthy weight is more important than simply being toned and sculpted. Right now, you just need to lose a little additional body fat; you can work on your abs later. People are attempting to play catch up and operate from a position of weakness as society becomes aware of what is occurring and that we are overweight as a culture. They want to live a healthy lifestyle and shed some pounds.

For many people, eating healthfully all the time feels prohibitively expensive and out of reach. Everyone would choose the appropriate foods if it didn't. But here's the thing: even if eating healthier can be difficult, it doesn't have to be. You just need to go through a little period of adjustment to find ways to make it simpler and more convenient.

This eBook will show you how to eat healthily and shed the first 10 pounds that so many of us find difficult to lose. It's remarkable how small adjustments to your daily routine, all of which center around healthy diet and regular exercise, may help you lose ten pounds.

**WARNING: Consult with a doctor or other appropriate professional before starting any diet, physical exercise program, or alteration to your regular habits.**

# CHAPTER 1

## QUIT EATING PROCESSED FOOD AND BEGIN DRINKING MORE WATER TO LOSE WEIGHT.

Simply stop eating manufactured foods and stop trying the trendy diets. Anything that has been processed, such as bags of chips, salty frozen meals, fast food, etc., will be packed with calories, chemicals, and salt.

Eating entire foods, such as fruits, vegetables, whole grains, and healthy fats, is preferable. Basically, the bulk of your diet should consist of anything you might grow or raise.

Put more consideration into it rather than mindlessly walking the grocery shop considering what you want to eat for the next one or two nights. Prepare a few meal ideas for the upcoming days before you go shopping, then put those products in your cart. This helps you succeed throughout the week by preventing you from purchasing harmful foods that you truly don't need.

People fail to recognize that the first step in shedding the initial 10 pounds is what they consume. In reality, most people are unaware that they may mistakenly believe they are hungry when they are truly dehydrated and actually thirsty. Water is marvelous. Your body weight is made up entirely of water, over 66%.

Water is essential for maintaining a healthy weight for the same reason.

Take in a lot of water. The suggested daily intake is eight glasses, although it can take you some time to get there. Your body need a ton of water. In addition to helping your body rid itself of impurities, water also improves your health and wellbeing. You just start to feel fit when you drink a lot of water, and this is the inspiration you need to slim down.

The nicest thing about water is that it has zero calories, so you may drink as much as you like. Because you won't feel as though you are starving to death when you drink a lot of water, you will also eat less. Always remember that if you feel hungry, you were probably simply thirsty and not at all hungry. Try drinking a glass of water first. The 8-glass recommendation each day is something you should aspire to. Purchasing a jug from the drugstore or grocery shop that is made to carry precisely 8 glasses of water is the easiest method to accomplish this and measure your water intake. These are fantastic tools for losing weight since you can fill them up, freeze them, and then have fresh, cold water all day as the ice melts. You can also drink your water at room temperature if you don't mind. It just matters that you are obtaining the water that your body need.

Obtain a glass of pure, fresh water to begin your day. Drink one as soon as you awaken in the morning. Your body won't have to struggle against dehydration, which will aid in its reactivation. Additionally, you won't need to have such a substantial breakfast after drinking a glass of water. All of your body's digestive juices are roused and thoroughly lubricated by a glass of water. You can always have your morning cup of coffee or tea, but remember to follow it up with a glass of water. You want to avoid becoming dehydrated since caffeine dehydrates you.

Before you start eating, sip on some water. Drinking water will help you feel fuller naturally, reducing the amount of food you need to eat.

Drink some water along with your meal. Drink something after every bite to help you feel filled without feeling bloated and to help you finish your meal more quickly. Additionally, drinking water as you eat will hasten the digestion of your food, causing you to experience fullness more rapidly.

Try your best to avoid drinking soda. All sodas are heavily sugar sweetened. It's best to eliminate as much of your diet as you can. Diet soda is still soda, too. Despite having less sugar, it still contains additional chemicals and ingredients that are bad for your health. When consuming soda, follow it up with a glass of water. Keep in mind that caffeine also dehydrates you. Sodas that have been decaffeinated still include small levels of caffeine and the same amount of sugar, making them not significantly healthier.

Juice made from fruits is not as nutritious as most people believe. Actually, juice contains a significant amount of sugar. Fresh fruit juice is preferable than juice with artificial flavors and coloring if you are seeking a glass of juice. If you can create your own fruit juice, that is even better. Just make careful to avoid adding too much sugar, which raises the calorie count. Eat more fruit rather than fruit juice. Fruit supplies your body with essential vitamins and fiber.

Don't drink too much coffee and tea. If you don't add a lot of cream and sugar to them, they are essentially safe. The cream and sugar turn into fatty ingredients. Consider it this way: Every time you drink a cup of coffee or tea with cream and two sugar cubes, it's like eating a piece of chocolate cake. Imagine how much cake you will consume after drinking a Starbucks Latte; ouch.

Try to only consume black tea and coffee if you absolutely must. As long as you drink plenty of water to balance your body's intake of caffeine after drinking black tea or coffee, there are health benefits. Because it alters bodily processes like your metabolism, caffeine is also bad for you.

Green tea is another variety of tea that you are free to consume. Thousands of years ago, green tea was utilized as medicinal in China. It supports the digestive system, can ease an excessively full stomach, and has been connected to a lower chance of developing cancer.

It is great if you are able to refuse alcohol. Although a glass of red wine does offer heart advantages, most alcoholic beverages are just fattening. Particularly fattening is beer. Depending on the ingredients they include, cocktails can make you fat. Take whiskey with Coke as an example. The Coke is undoubtedly fatty, but the whiskey might not be. Additionally, most people have the munchies after a few drinks, and when you're a little tipsy and hungry, you won't be able to make sane decisions about your diet. It's also common to overeat in the late evening, right before you pass out following a night of drinking. Simply put, the entire mix is poor.

If alcohol is a must, try dry wine. Due to the higher sugar content in sweet wines, dry wine is preferable. Although dry wines do contain sugar, the majority of it has been fermented into alcohol, making them healthier for weight gain.

One more thing about coffee: it's not always bad, but it's more intriguing than anything. Some claim that they shed more weight when they drank black coffee before working out. Nutritionists speculate that it might be brought on by the body being pushed to use fat as fuel, however there is no scientific evidence to support this. Hey, if you can handle black coffee, it's worth a go. Just keep in mind to stay hydrated while working out!

To prevent your body from becoming desensitized to caffeine's natural fat-burning properties, limit your coffee consumption. If the day is particularly slow to start, no more than one or two cups.

Remember, avoid shopping when you're hungry to avoid buying all the snacks.

# CHAPTER 2

## BE REALISTIC: EAT WELL TO LOSE WEIGHT

Be realistic about your goals and expectations if you're transitioning from not eating well to eating well. Don't go into this expecting to completely change everything right away. It may take some time for you to adjust, and it's fine if you "fail" and don't eat super healthy every day. It's more about finding a happy medium than being "perfect."

Set small goals, lower your expectations, and give yourself permission to do your best under the circumstances. Even if you don't realize it right away, relieving stress will make things easier.

Alright, when most individuals consider losing weight while eating, they consider dieting. Unluckily, the majority of popular diets today tend to make people gain weight. Why? due to the fact that they starve them till they pass out and when this happens, the victim eventually succumbs to their hunger and consumes everything in sight. Furthermore, they deny them their favorite foods. Both weight loss and daily living cannot be accomplished in this manner. You only harm yourself by putting yourself under stress, which makes you eat more.

So, there are a few dietary guidelines you can adhere to every day that won't prevent you from enjoying the foods you love but will instead consider them as luxuries that will increase your enjoyment of them.

You will feel fuller for a longer amount of time if you eat foods high in protein and fiber. You're less likely to grab for junk food the rest of the day if you eat meals and snacks full of these ingredients. Excellent sources of protein include eggs, lean meats, poultry, and beans. You may get the necessary fiber from fruits, vegetables, and nuts.

Obtain your daily servings of fresh produce with a high-water content. These include items such as tomatoes, watermelons, cantaloupe, kiwi, grapes, etc. All of those luscious, fresh fruits and vegetables are healthy for you. Since these foods are between 90 and 95 percent water, you can eat a lot of them and they won't make you gain weight. Replace processed fruit with fresh fruit. anything that is converted into additional sugar. Fruits that have been processed or canned likewise lack the fiber that fresh fruits possess. As much as you can, increase your intake of fiber. Typically, this entails consuming more fruits and vegetables.

When it comes to losing weight, vegetables are your friends. There are many options available here, and you might even wish to try ones that you haven't tried before. The greatest types of greens are leafy, and you should always incorporate salads into your meals when you can. As long as you don't drown them in cheese and excessive dressing, salads are nutrient-rich meals. There is a lot of natural water in the leafy greens as well.

Think carefully about your food choices. Eat just when you are hungry. Animals eat out of instinct, but humans only eat when they are aware that their bodies are truly hungry. Avoid impulsive eating.
 Pay attention to everything you eat, from the dish itself to the toppings. Because they are frequently heavy in fat, garnishes and condiments can ruin a balanced dinner.

Control your sweet tooth, you can still enjoy your favorite treats as long as you don't eat them as a meal. Always keep in mind that these treats contribute to a region that you don't want them to contribute to. However, don't starve yourself either because you'll eat twice as much as you should if you do.

Establish and adhere to mealtimes, try to schedule your meals so that you can consume them at those times. You can manage when and what you eat by developing an eating routine. Additionally, eating five little meals throughout the day is preferable to just one or two large ones. Your body feels as though it is famished when you only eat once a day, which causes it to store fat rather than use it as fuel. Do not wait until you are famished before eating. You will only eat excessively till full as a result of this. Only eat when you are truly hungry. Make careful to first sip on some water to ascertain whether you are truly thirsty or truly hungry. It's common for people to eat when they see food. They simply want to consume it; it does not imply that they are hungry. If you're not truly hungry, don't accept any food that is offered to you. If you feel obligated to eat it out of politeness, simply nibble; skip a meal.

Try to avoid snacking in between meals, but if you must, make sure it is a healthy snack. If you travel frequently, try to select healthy snacks rather than fast food. Vegetables are excellent snacks, If you are experiencing hunger pangs, they can help you get through them. Because they are nutrient-rich and satiate hunger, carrots are wonderful.

For those foods that must be consumed, counting calories is a good idea. If the food is packed, the calories will be listed on the packaging. Make careful to consider the caloric content of serving sizes as well. Because an Otis Spunkmeyer muffin is meant to be two servings, you must multiply the calorie count by two. Here is where food producers start to play shady, and you must not fall for their tricks.

By the end of the week, burn off the excess calories. Make sure to visit the gym or go for a longer walk if you feel like you have indulged excessively this week in order to burn off those additional calories. Avoid anything that has been fried. It is preferable to bake anything that has been breaded. Foods that are fried are covered in fat and oil. Even after the extra oil has been removed, oil is still absorbed into the food item. Avoid skipping meals, A minimum of three meals each day are recommended, but five small meals are preferred. As a result, you won't become ravenous during the day and end up overeating.

Fresh vegetables are preferable to canned ones, much like fruits. If you can eat your vegetables raw, that is even better. The nutrients are lost when you cook them. If you must cook them, try to boil them just long enough to keep some of their crispness. Don't dunk them in butter either. It would be best if you could purchase organic vegetables free of pesticides.

Limit your egg consumption to one per day. The best option is to limit your egg consumption to three per week. Treating chocolates as a luxury is appropriate. Purchase quality products, and consume them infrequently. Each bite will taste even better if you actually take the time to appreciate it. You'll also enjoy eating them more.

Every day, eat items from all the food groups. This is a fantastic technique to make sure you are getting all the nutrients your body need and it aids in preventing any dietary deficits. Additionally, avoid eating the same things repeatedly. Try new things to avoid getting bored with your current diet. If possible, try to have breakfast an hour after waking up. The greatest method to give your body the boost it needs is to do this. Avoid waiting till you are genuinely hungry.

Although breakfast is crucial, you shouldn't overeat. You're supposed to be breaking your fast after not eating all night.

All food groups, including carbs, should be present in your diet. Your diet should consist of 50–55 percent carbohydrates. A significant source of energy is carbs. Diets that forbid carbs are harmful to you and just increase your cravings for them. You shouldn't lack any nutrients due to your diet. Your diet should only contain 25 to 30 percent protein. The idea that meat should be the focal point of your meal is overemphasized. In reality, it is more appropriate to classify it as a side dish as opposed to the main meal.

Your lunch should contain 15–25% fat. This is all the fat your body actually need. You'll be eating a lot of this in the diet in the form of cream, sugar, and other things. consume more white than red meat. Chicken, fish, and some other poultry are examples of white flesh. Beef and pork are examples of red meat.

As much as you can, try to eat vegetarian. Even if you can't entirely cut out meat, this is still a better way of living. The better is to consume as many fruits and vegetables as you can. The more meat you eliminate from your diet, the more fat you may eliminate as well. However, protein is crucial, so be sure your choice enables you to maintain healthy protein levels.

White bread is good, but multigrain breads high in fiber are considerably superior. These breads provide a good amount of protein and are another option to increase your diet's fiber intake. In no way does eating pork help you lose weight. When attempting to lose weight, it is best to consume less pork. Foods like bacon, ham, and sausage are made from pork, which also has a high fat content. Consume sugar as little as possible. If you must sweeten your coffee and tea, look for an artificial sweetener whose flavor you enjoy. However, these activities should also be restricted because they are not particularly healthy either.

Attempt to graze five to six times daily. These are the snacks that we previously spoke about. Some people find that they lose weight more successfully when they never feel hungry, and you can achieve this by grazing on healthy foods. Additionally, it keeps your metabolism active, which naturally burns fat. Do not worry about cheating, but avoid doing so during meals. Eat desserts and your preferred cheat food just for the flavor. After dinner, if you want dessert, split one with your entire family. You won't gain weight, only flavor.

Watch your consumption of fat. A gram of fat contains 9 calories. You can calculate the quantity of fat in those things if you know your overall calorie intake. Try to use half as much salt as you normally would and go gentle on it. One of the biggest contributors to obesity is salt.

CHAPTER 3

## CHANGING YOUR COOKING PROCESS TO LOSE WEIGHT AND KEEPING YOUR KITCHEN STOCKED

Simply removing harmful items from your kitchen is one method to reduce the temptation to eat them. Throw away any bags of cookies or chips that you want to get rid of, and stock up on healthier alternatives in their place. Stock your refrigerator with plenty of fruits, vegetables, yogurts, and other wholesome foods. For the pantry, purchase wholesome snack alternatives. You're more likely to feed your body the proper foods if the right foods are readily available in your kitchen.

Prepare and cook breakfast, lunch, and dinner, or at least some of them, throughout the course of one half-day. Stock the refrigerator after separating each meal into a separate container. During the week, you may quickly cook one up if you're hungry yet pressed for time.

Here are a few pointers that will enable you to drop the first ten pounds by just altering your diet preparation. Food's nutritional value is equally dependent on how it is prepared.

Try baking those items rather of deep-frying them in lard or oil. The amount of grease and oil used for baking is less than that needed for frying, and the dish does not absorb up those ingredients while it cooks. To avoid using oil, spray non-stick cooking pans. Additionally, non-stick pans require little to no oil at all. Instead of frying, boil your vegetables.

The healthiest method to consume veggies like cabbage, cauliflower, broccoli, and carrots is probably to steam them, so you can do that as well.

Foods with no or little fat should be avoided. These food products are widely available, although they are not particularly healthful. Many of these foods are sweetened with a chemical or carbohydrate to improve their flavor. These substances and carbohydrates are nevertheless converted by the body into sugar, which implies that fat is still formed from them. Avoid being a diet crasher. These are unhealthy and ultimately cause more harm than benefit. Usually, you will drop a few pounds in the short term, but once you stop, everything returns, and your weight gets worse. Crash diets are impossible to maintain, and ultimately you have to stop.

Regardless of whether it is liquid meal, dessert, or ice cream, chew it at least 8 to 12 times. Saliva is added to the food, aiding in the sugar's digestion. When food isn't thoroughly chewed and is instead just swallowed, you flood your stomach with undigestible food that doesn't provide the necessary health advantages. Use high-quality extra virgin olive oil when cooking. It is more expensive than vegetable oil, but because of the superior health advantages, the price is justified. Olive oil helps to strengthen the suppleness of the arterial walls, which lowers the risk of heart attack and stroke. It has also been linked to a lower risk of coronary heart disease.

CHAPTER 4

# WORKOUT TO LOSE WEIGHT

You need to do two things in order to lose weight, and one of them—eating healthy foods and drinking lots of pure water—has already been discussed in great detail here. Get your body moving as another requirement. For the purpose of exercising, you don't need to join a gym. In truth, there are a number of daily activities you may engage in to help your body start losing weight, as well as a number of workouts you can undertake alone to accomplish so.

Don't give up when you start exercising, whether it's at home or in a gym, if you don't notice results right away. To start improving and getting your body into shape, it takes longer than a week. Many people make the error of thinking that their exercise is ineffective when it only requires a brief period of time.

When you initially start exercising, injuries may result from pushing your body too far. Your ligaments, joints, and bones are not designed to withstand the strain you are placing on them. Do not believe that if you really push yourself during a few workouts that you will lose money; sadly, this is not how the body functions. In terms of exercise, slow and steady is better than fast and furious. When you first begin exercising, weigh yourself, but don't use it as a gauge for your weight loss. Your weight changes during the course of the day.

If you weigh yourself every day, you might simply end up giving up. The fit of your garments is the best indicator of weight loss. You'll know that eating right and exercise are helping you if you start to feel like you're floating around in your clothes. Moving where you normally fasten your belt—tighter is obviously better—is another sign that you're losing weight.

Reward yourself when you regularly check your weight and the way your clothes fit. Purchase a new pair of pants or a new pair of running shoes for yourself. As you work toward your weight loss objectives, this will support you in staying motivated.

Give your body a day off from exercise so it can recuperate and heal itself. Every week, your body requires a day off. In order to start losing weight, you need at least four days of 30-minute activity, and five days a week is much better. Three days of 30-minute exercise will help you maintain your weight.

Gather information about simple activities you may perform at home and about exercise. There is a ton of in-depth research on exercise accessible, and you may choose what will help you the most to achieve your weight loss objectives. For further information on how to burn the target number of calories you want to burn each week, browse the web or have a look at some books on health and fitness that are available at your local library or bookstore.

In search of a workout partner, the person you choose for this should share your commitment to exercise and weight loss. Finding a devoted relationship has its benefits, including the ability to provide you someone to feel accountable to. You find it easier to get out of bed and join someone for exercise when you know they are waiting for you. Your exercise partner is someone you wouldn't want to stand up. Take a rest when your body signals that it has had enough. You will begin to feel messages from your body once you have exercised for a while. When you are just beginning your fitness regimen, this is especially crucial. Do it gradually if you desire to lengthen your workouts. Your workout intensity is exactly the same.

Choose a workout plan that complements your lifestyle. Everyone has a distinct lifestyle and works in a different field. There is no specific time that you must or must not exercise. If you find that working out late before bed is calming for you, then do it. It's also fantastic if you prefer to exercise first thing in the morning because it helps you wake up. Due to the stress of their jobs or because it is the only time they have available, some people like working out during their lunch break. Instead of standing still, move around. Do it if you can move around. Pacers actually benefit greatly from their frequent movement since it helps them stay healthy. You can think better through pacing.

If you are able to stand, do so. If you can stand without discomfort, standing burns more calories than sitting does. When you can sit, avoid lying down. similar to the first two in idea.

The couch and the TV are detrimental to losing weight. Don't sit on it if you have a tendency to turn into a couch potato. To avoid wasting too much time in front of the television, if necessary, place a less comfortable chair there. If you're a computer addict, the same applies to that device. Some people find that sitting in front of their computer is more comfortable than sitting in front of the television. (This is, of course, if you don't work from home and must sit in front of a computer for extended periods of time, in which case your chair is crucial.) At least every half an hour, get up and stretch if your job requires you to sit all day. Today's occupations mostly need you to sit down in front of a computer. Make it a point to relocate occasionally if your job is one like this.

While you're on the phone, move around. If the chat is lengthy, you'll get a nice workout. Take the stairs rather than the escalator or elevator. Despite being wonderful conveniences, these things make us exceedingly lazy. Additionally, taking the stairs can be quicker than waiting for an elevator to open.

Don't smoke. Smoking does not directly cause weight gain, but it does cause unpredictable eating patterns and increases caffeine dependence. Most people should obtain 10 minutes of cardio each day, and there are alternatives to running for this. Try 15 minutes of brisk walking to stay fit if you are physically unable to run. If you have the time, you can walk everywhere. Consider biking or walking if your place of employment or the grocery store is nearby. Even though it might take a little longer, you'll still be exercising.

Avert your own eyes by hiding the remote. As far as weight loss is concerned, remote controllers are equally bad. In the absence of a remote, you might not even turn on the television, which suggests that you might look for more engaging activities to perform. If you don't have a remote, get up and change the station, or take a walk instead of watching TV. Make your own fetching. You should walk and get it yourself if you need something from the kitchen, the TV station changed, the mail, or the newspaper from the driveway. You will benefit much from increasing your daily walking.

During commercials, you can either move around or perform easy workouts like crunches or bending over and touching your toes. Do whatever it takes to keep your blood circulating and your body moving. Play some music, and start moving. It goes without saying that the more you move, the better you'll feel and the more weight you'll shed. Get off a block before your stop if you're taking public transportation, then continue walking. Using this method, you can fit in walks before and after work or on the way to somewhere else.

To tone your midsection, perform pelvic gyrations. These are obviously inappropriate to perform in public, but they are an excellent first step in preparing your body for more challenging stomach crunches. Additionally, it helps your back muscles and keeps you relaxed rather than tight. Walk with a suck in your stomach. Keep your stomach tucked in when walking appropriately. Those muscles will start to stiffen up soon. Toning your midriff requires breathing workouts. It is incredible how using your entire diaphragm to breathe properly can actually aid to strengthen your abdominal muscles. Since oxygen is good for the brain, most individuals already breathe too little.

Try out some yoga. Yoga is a fantastic stress-reduction and weight-loss method. Yoga teaches you how to regulate your muscles and increase your control over the many muscle groups that make up your body. Carry weights. People underestimate the amount of fat that strength training can burn. When you work on developing muscle, your body starts to burn fat as fuel for your growing muscles. Be aware that because muscle weighs more than fat, your scale might not accurately reflect your weight loss as you add muscle. Petrify your lover. If they have been working out with you, you can exert a little while also congratulating them on the weight they have shed.

# CHAPTER 5

## LOSE WEIGHT AND KEEP IT OFF

Here is some additional advice on how to lose weight and keep it off, and it all starts with what you eat.

We are bigger than ever, making weight loss and being overweight such a crucial part of our lives nowadays. Anyone listening in on a discussion or watching television will be drawn in when they hear the phrase "weight loss programs." In fact, one of the most frequently searched keywords on the Internet right now is that.

Our relationship with food is the fundamental explanation of why we are so overweight. In our culture, we frequently place an emphasis on quantity. Instead of the best cuisine available, we simply want as much as we can obtain. When it should be the exact opposite, quantity always triumphs over quality.

It might be challenging to decide where to start once you've made the decision to reduce weight. It is achievable if you have a strong desire to start working out and lose weight. You simply need to learn how to refuse requests.

Each person is unique. You won't come across anyone else who has the same metabolism as you or burns fat in the same manner. Even if you both started an exercise and nutrition program the same way every day and had the exact same weight, you and the person next to you might not have the same outcomes two weeks or even a month later. While this is true, it's vital to keep in mind that not everyone uses food in the same way. What might make one individual gain a pound might not have the same effect on another.  Weight loss follows the same rules. Even if you eat the same foods and exercise in the same ways, you and your husband might not experience the same results if you're a married woman working out with him. For example, if he stops drinking soda and loses five pounds as a result, but you lose only one, that proves that you and your husband might not experience the same results.

The fact is that modern society requires much more effort than earlier cultures did. Because they had to work, both men and women were skinny sixty years ago. It was necessary to perform manual labor in order to have access to food. For fresh milk, you had to go milk the cows, and if you wanted vegetables, you had to plough the fields. If you wanted eggs, you had to go get them from the hen house. If you wanted meat, you had to be aware of the process of growing a calf and having it killed. That was how things were back then, and technology has eliminated all of this laborious labor.  As a result, we must monitor our diet and force ourselves to exercise. If we don't, half the time we have no cause to move.

It is crucial to realize that your ability to work hard toward your weight loss objectives will determine how successful you are. It's the one thing you need to work hard for in life to get if you want to see results.

Typically, people do not have to worry about weight loss until they are in their twenties, but with the prevalence of fast food in our culture today, this is not always the case. Due to their excessive consumption of processed foods and fast food, many of our youngsters are obese. When you go grocery shopping for yourself and your family, check the labels on the food you will be consuming. Don't consume something if you can't say its name. Processed foods make us crave unhealthy foods, which makes us gain weight. If you want to ever be successful at losing weight and keeping it off, it is very crucial that you grasp this.

However, merely monitoring your diet won't result in weight loss. The right diet must be combined with the right volume of exercise. The answer is to follow an exercise routine that will provide your body with the workout it needs to burn calories and fat effectively. If you don't move around, it's as though you're in hibernation and your body just continues to put on weight, especially around your waist.

It just makes you feel nice all over when you recall a time when the sun and hard work were the causes of your sweat. You feel stronger all over as a result of the sun's direct impact on your shoulders and the tension it places on your muscles.

Working out outside is the best thing there is.

However, the majority of people now live in cities. For the most part, the days of working on a farm are long gone, but for a small number of people, the joy of working and creating something tangible while also maintaining their weight loss is still available. Consider how many farm workers, cowboys, and ranchers there are; how many of them are obese. Not a lot of them exist. Just imagine how they live.  They rise, take a cup of coffee, eat breakfast, leave for work, return for lunch, return for dinner, and then go to bed early enough to get up the next morning and repeat the process all over again. They enjoy all-day access to fresh water, good sunlight, and clean air in the meantime. This way of life is really healthy. The majority of us work indoors, sitting down, and regrettably, we still eat three meals a day, but we have to rush through it so you don't even get a chance to taste it.

Except for those who live in cities where they can walk everywhere, it is a fact of life that city dwellers don't get much exercise. This implies that you must work hard and set your mind to it. You must incorporate exercise into your everyday routine to avoid being overweight and ill. It simply so happens that way. Exercise is the best approach to treat obesity, stress, hypertension, cardio vascular disease, and other disorders linked to a sedentary lifestyle. Better still if you can work out outside. As much clean air as you can get is what your body needs.

The most crucial component of any fitness program is consistency. You can achieve your goals if you set them and continually work toward them.

Most people find it simple to start. They go shopping, purchase some activewear, running shoes, and perhaps a gym membership. After that, they engage in fairly consistent exercise for a week or two.

However, they find it more difficult to stick to their regimen as they proceed. Their daily obligations increase, and they start going to the gym less frequently. In other words, they simply quit attending to the gym after their subscription is wasted.

Even though many people prefer to exercise in the evenings, other people find it more difficult to stick with this schedule. This is an excellent time to leave if you are not entirely worn out when you get off work. However, if you are unable to, you might need to figure out a way to travel there in the morning. You'll be able to stay consistent and it will assist you get awake.

Contrary to popular belief, exercise doesn't always leave you feeling exhausted. It might affect you in this way at first, but as you get fitter, you'll notice that you have more energy. You shouldn't have any trouble getting up in the morning and getting going if you combine exercise with enough sleep. Additionally, you'll be energized the entire day, which will make it lot simpler for you to get through your job.

There's a good chance that your home has a sidewalk and some people might even have access to a pool, even if you don't have a gym membership. Get up 30 minutes early, put on your sneakers, and start your preferred kind of exercise, such as walking or running. Pets will undoubtedly enjoy spending time with you over this period if you have any.

All this illustrates how walking is a fantastic form of exercise and weight loss. Walking is an excellent place to start if you're too busy to work out.

Below you'll find some useful information on the calories we burn when we exercise.

| Exercise | Calories Burned |
| --- | --- |
| Aerobics | 200-250 |
| Stationary Bicycling | 250-300 |
| Actual Bicycling | 300-400 |
| Running | 300-350 |
| Stair climbing | 200-250 |
| Swimming Laps | 350 |
| Brisk Walking | 150-180 |
| Cultivating Your Garden | 130-200 |
| Sex (Yes, sex is another form of exercise too) | 50-60 |
| Playing Basketball | 130-250 |
| Golf – carrying clubs, no cart | 166 |
| Water Skiing | 180-200 |
| Ice Skating – general | 200-250 |
| General Skiing | 200-250 |

**CHAPTER 6**

# FASTING: INTERMITTENT

What is meant exactly by intermittent fasting? Fasting is a term that almost everyone is familiar with. Each group has its own unique set of motivations for fasting. Some people sacrifice food as part of their religious rituals in order to dedicate themselves to prayer. Some individuals are hungry for no apparent cause. People used to go out into the fields to work and would only eat when they were taking a break.

Among the above-mentioned fasting methods, intermittent fasting is not one of them. It is a decision rather than a religious practice or a result of a lack of time or food. It can best be described as a pattern of eating that alternates between eating and fasting times, with each time lasting a specific amount of time. For instance, the 16:8 technique calls for 16 hours of fasting and 8 hours of eating.

Be aware that it is an eating pattern rather than a diet. Less is said about the items you should eat, but timing is more stressed. Does this imply that you can eat whatever you want? Sadly, no. You will get out of life what you put into it, just like anything else. One of the three components of the tripod for successful weight loss is clean eating. Does this imply that you must subsist solely on chicken and broccoli? No, of course not. Since we are all human, I think it is important to enjoy life, but as you are already aware, moderation is the key in this situation.

It is important to know that IF isn't some program that popped up from somewhere, will trend for a while, and disappear like most weight loss programs do. It has been around for a long time and has been popular for many years (even if you are learning about it just now). It is one of the leading health and fitness trends in the world today.

Researchers have tested intermittent fasting and shown it to be an effective weight loss and fat-burning strategy. But exactly how does it operate? Prior to learning how IF functions, it's crucial to comprehend the following points:

How the body uses energy and how it is stored

Your hormones' function in this procedure

Either the body is conserving energy or it is burning it. There is no room for compromise.

Why does this matter? In general, if you don't burn glucose (sugar), you either store it as glycogen or fat. Does this imply that you should exercise regularly? Simple reply: No. Exercise actually only accounts for 10%–15% of the weight loss equation (more about that later). Your body uses a variety of distinct processes to burn energy. Your body uses energy even while you're standing still and doing nothing since it needs to carry out necessary processes to keep you alive. RMR or BMR both refer to this. Your cells might use glucose and burn it for energy, but any extra will be stored.

Wait! Logically, eating less and exercising more would result in weight loss if we were either storing sugar or burning it. Right, it looks simple enough. Most are, if you're reading this, you've already tried this strategy without success. Either you started to see benefits only to have them abruptly stop, or you gained it all back once you resumed your regular way of living.

How then do I lose weight? We must comprehend two concepts in order to have a clearer picture:

How glucose (sugar) is retained, burnt, or utilized as an energy source.

Our hormones' function in this procedure

In what way is energy kept? Glycogen and fat are two different ways the body can store energy. Digestion converts food (yum) into a range of distinct macronutrients. The bloodstream carries these macronutrients to our cells where they are used for a variety of bodily processes. For instance, carbohydrates are converted to glucose (sugar), which is then absorbed by the bloodstream and delivered to cells for use as fuel. But if there is too much glucose in the blood (high blood sugar), it will be turned into glycogen through a process known as glycogenesis. Glycogen has a maximum amount the body can store. Any surplus glucose is then stored as fat through a process known as lipogenesis after these stores are full.

How is energy utilized?

Glycogen undergoes a process known as glycogenolysis in order to convert back into glucose when our cells need more energy than the bloodstream can supply (low blood sugar). In order to return our blood sugar levels to normal, our glycogen reserves are gradually depleted. When these reserves run out, a process known as lipolysis will break down fat for energy. We're now burning fat.

There is a lot to be talked about in this subject that helps you lose weight. The full explanation of how fasting helps to achieve your desired result. That will be talked more about in my book on fasting. Titled 'FASTING AND WEIGHT LOSE'

There are many ways you can burn fat; just search for the exercise you can do to achieve this.

Thanks for reading my book, if you have any question on anything pertaining to this subject, please feel free to e-mail me mirrow007@gmail.com I will be waiting to respond.

# ABOUT THE AUTHOR

"Jerry Efe Xavier Osagie popularly called "Jex Xavier" has been an IT and multimedia expert, creative designer and teacher." My personal growth journey made me aware of how crucial it is to have specific goals. Surprisingly, few people have objectives that motivate them to get out of bed in the morning, and even fewer have specific, written goals that they are working on every day. That epiphany inspired me to write this book. Because I genuinely believe that what we do every day influences what we'll achieve in life, I decided to write about habits. Ironically, it took me a lot of failures before I ultimately developed the practice of making goals each day. Setting goals has turned out to be its own habit, and without it, I never would have produced the book you're currently reading.